asphyxiation

a novella

by Susan Black

WINDSOR HOUSE
PUBLISHING GROUP INC.

Windsor House Publishing Group
Salt Lake City, Utah

asphyxiation

In association with Woodward Books

SOON TO BE A MAJOR MOTION PICTURE

This is a work of fiction.
All characters and events portrayed in this book are fictional,
and any resemblance to real people or incidents is purely coincidental.

For information address: Windsor House Publishing Group
73 West Plumtree Lane, Suite 13F, Salt Lake City, Utah 84047

PRINTING HISTORY
First Printing 1996

ISBN: 1-881636-08-9

Books are published by Windsor House Publishing Group, Incorporated,
73 West Plumtree Lane, Suite 13F, Salt Lake City, Utah 84047.
The name "Windsor House" and the logo are trademarks belonging to
Windsor House Publishing Group, Incorporated.

PRINTED IN THE UNITED STATES OF AMERICA.
10 9 8 7 6 5 4 3 2 1

for Wendy

and Cindy

the Sleepy Beauty

and all the Norma Jeans

Author's Acknowledgements

With love and thanks to those who believed:

LB, Bet and Bill, Kathy and Ricky, Dot and Jim, Dot and Jack,
Doyal and Martha, Helen, K & M, M & M, Sarah and Derek,
Syd and Marilyn, Amy & gals, Rita, Diana and Kevin,
Pat and Jay, JM & Liz, Char and Bob, Baker, Ed, KJ, Duncan and Catherine,
Jean, Dave B, Cherri, Anne, Stephan, Kim, Jim and Suzy, Big Daddy & L,
JB, John, Jess, Stephanie, Luke, Lea, Brett, Barry,
Joshua Brand and John Falsey, Karen and Barbara Hall, J. M. Straczynski,
John Marsh, Colin Callender, Karith, Jay, Lesli Linka,
Cathy Konrad, Pat Saphier, Mike Kappus, Father Kaiser,
Judith Guest,
Louise Fletcher,
The New York Writer's Foundation,
Woodward Books,
The American Film Institute,
all the adults who took time to read to me

and

The Boys for taking the risk
Ted for removing the blinders

and

The Clay Man for helping me rediscover the path

.........*one*

Blackness envelops a woman's bored voice.

"Eye contact."

Darting pupil, restless eye reflects a flickering neon motel sign that has seen far better days.

She sighs as if inhaling an entire century.

"That's the whole damn problem."

.... *two*

"Hey there."

The man leans on the bar. Staring.

Alex keeps drinking. Pointed black cowboy boots at ease on the barstool. Short skirt riding legs that have been places. Eyes straight ahead. Captivating.

"How about I buy you a drink?"

He sits.

Alex keeps staring back at her past.

"I have a drink."

"Have another one."

He signals Ray, the burly bartender.

"Where you from? That accent is ferociously sexy."

Alex sips methodically, mind adrift.

"You have a name?"

Alex still stares. In the light she looks like another Marilyn.

"Do you?" She relishes the retort. It only makes him smile.

"Frank."

"Frank what?"

He leans into her ear. A slushy whisper.

"Frank Campbell."

Alex slowly turns. Smiles into his face. Lips almost touching.

"Frank Campbell, your ex-wife's been looking for you." A subpoena slaps in his face.

"Damn!"

"You oughta be ashamed Frank. Not paying that child support."

She puts down money. Eyes smiling at Ray.

"I love it when you do that, Alex." Ray watches her. Wistful.

"Night, Ray." Black boots disappear out the door.

Frank just stares. An empty glass.

.... *three*

The '55 Cadillac insignia glints off the dying sun. Siren Red fingernails flip on the radio and crank up pumping music. Deafening.

A Marilyn Monroe air freshener flaps on the dash. Taped in a moment of inspiration lifetimes ago.

The tires hug the curves. Too fast. Squealing.

The convertible silhouette pulls into the searing sunset. Black boots rest in the dirt. Lost against the desert sky.

Silence.

Alex breathes.

.........*four*

Streetlights illuminate the Cadillac insignia. No longer awash in a dying sun. The headlights turn off outside the cozy house.

Sit. Waiting.

A light in the window of the house. Suddenly.

Restless fingers, red nails, hold a dying cigarette.

Alex stares ahead at nothing. Doesn't get out.

Can't.

Inside, half-shaven Matt sulks in a house robe, watching the dark silhouette in front of the house. Willing her inside.

The cigarette burns low. She ejects it out the window. Her last excuse at staying in the dark.

Pulls herself out of the car towards the house.

A disapproving glance from Matt at the door.

"Norma Jean couldn't sleep. Wanted to know when her Mama was comin' home."

Alex sweeps Norma Jean into her arms. Both light at each other's smile. Alex strokes the honey colored hair.

"Hi, baby."

Matt moves toward her. Alex brushes past him up the stairs. Hesitates at the painting dominating the hallway. Bride. Groom. Picket fence. He watches her sigh uncomfortably at his creation.

Escape into Norma's room.

"Where'd you go?" Norma's face wrinkles in a question.

"Sometimes I just....need.....to.....watch a sunset."

Norma searches her face.

"Why?"

Alex swallows the tears. Manages a smile.

"I don't know, baby." She sighs at the kaleidoscope of colors in the room. "I just do."

Matt cuts a hurt look at the present sitting on Alex's bed. Unopened. Grabs his keys. Past her portrait. Elusive as the wind.

Covers tuck around the angel face. Lips brush the innocent forehead.

"Close your eyes. It's late."

Eyes close. Eyes open.

"You'll be here in the morning?" A plaintive plea.

Alex smiles at her creation. Her hope.

"Ssssh. Mama's here."

The truck door slams outside. Guns into the night.

Headlights flash against baby doll wallpaper. Disappear with a squeal.

Darkness again. Another sigh.

"Mama's always here, baby."

.........*five*

The present in the shadows on a chair. Still unwrapped.

Alex's tousled hair buried in the pillows. Restless dreams.

A shaft of light from the hallway.

Matt staggers in. Stares at Alex. An alcohol daze.

Weaves to the bed. A burning hand on her thigh. She pushes it away.

"I need you…Allie."

Her eyes open. Troubled.

"Needin' got us Norma. Got us here."

The sober truth hangs in the darkness between them.

He sinks to his knees. Buries his head on her stomach.

"You're my…angel…Allie. I need you. Like that night… you first looked at me. Like that, Allie. Please."

His sobs shake them both. She closes her eyes. Rubs his head. Like a child.

"Matt…"

"Whatever I did, I'm sorry. I'm sorry. Please…" He raises his eyes. Pleading. "Please just let me…Touch you. If I don't… I'll…disappear."

Alex cups his face. Gently.

"Look at me, Matt. Look at me hard."

She wipes his tear. He pulls her legs around him.

She doesn't resist.

"There's no such thing." Her lips brush his face with regret. "Angels."

He kisses her.
Smother.

.........six

Morning. Eyes flutter open. Stare at the ceiling.

Suffocating.

The present leers at Alex. Alone.

She pulls off the lid. Doesn't touch the exquisite perfume bottle.

An angel in flight.

.... *seven*

A stoplight turns red. The Cadillac pulls up to it.

Alex lights a cigarette. Norma Jean plays with the pack. Spills a few.

"Put those away, baby." She takes them from Norma. Norma scowls. Precocious.

"Daddy doesn't like you smoking, Mama."

A sigh. "Lots o' things Daddy doesn't like, baby."

A sportscar revs up beside. The handsome driver smiles. Norma Jean watches him. The man smiles again. Devours Alex with his eyes.

Alex smiles back. Eyes sure.

The light turns green.

"Mama, that man's smiling at you. Who is he, Mama?"

Black boots gun the accelerator. Hard to resist.

"Trouble. He's just trouble, baby."

The Cadillac squeals through the light. Alex looks in the rearview. Trouble looks good.

"He's a stranger, Mama. 'Never talk to strangers.'"

The sportscar catches up, holds Alex's speed. She smiles again. "I didn't talk to him. I smiled at him."

The sportscar disappears into the afternoon.

The Cadillac pulls up to Norma's school. Alex watches a little girl, overdressed. With makeup. She smears on lipstick.

Norma bolts out. "Why'd you smile at him, Mama?"

"I don't know, baby. Felt nice. Give me a hug."

Norma hugs her and skips off. "Read with me later."

Alex leans her chin on the car door. Watches the little boy pinch the made-up girl. "Okay, baby."

The lipstick drops.

Clunk.

.... *eight*

Alex looks at the pathetic stack of legal documents in the District Attorney's courthouse office. Bored.

"Hey, Mike, this it?"

Mike, a hippie Assistant D.A. yells from inside his office. "Yeah."

"Shit." Alex lights a cigarette. "Do me a favor, Mike. Pay me a salary. This amounts to about a nickel."

Mike shuffles out of his tomb. "Can I help it if nothing vermicious happens in the summer?"

"Vermicious? You must have court today. Who you practicing those big words for?"

"Judge Meyer. Assault."

Alex sighs. Looks out past the sleepy town. "God, summer used to mean...more than being too damn hot..."

"Don't worry, Alex, in the fall, everybody'll be back from vacation, mad as hell, suing each other, things'll pick up."

She sucks on her cigarette. Somewhere else.

Mike watches her mouth. Lips working the end of the cigarette. "Hey, you okay?"

Outside an old couple scream at each other. Arguing. Alex watches them, pockets the documents to serve total strangers. "Sure, Mike. Same as always." Looks at him for the first time. "Anybody interesting?"

"Pissed off landlords. Matrimonial bliss. Same old stuff. Love does make the world go round now, don't it?"

She pulls the gun from her belt. Checks it comfortably.

Mike cringes. "Jesus, Alex. Do you mind?"

Alex smiles. "Afraid I'll shoot you?"

Mike dials the phone. "Don't take any shit on your rounds. Jimmy got a crowbar in the ribs from one of those house fraus."

Alex turns to go. Mike watches her hips maneuver. She tosses words at him without looking. "Jimmy probably asked for it."

.........*nine*

Black boots step over a man clutching a wine bottle. Crunch crack vials.

A graffiti door. Alex pushes through.

Someone whistles at her.

Inside the tenement, Alex passes bullets in the plaster. Muffled TVs drone. Something smells sour.

Alex's heart pumps. Sweat. The rush of confrontation. She puts a hand on the gun in her belt. Ready.

A loud noise suddenly punctures the surreal world. Alex turns and shoots in one fluid movement. Without hesitation.

An overturned trashcan rolls aimlessly. A mammoth rat lies in its own blood. Beady eyes. Glassy.

Alex stares at it. Eyes lit.

She moves past another door. More graffiti.

Finally knocks.

A woman appears. Burnt out.

"Francis Rodriguez?" Alex tries to look beyond the woman's pain.

The woman ignores the crying baby she holds. A toddler clings to her, eyes wide. Afraid of the stranger.

"What's he done now?" she asks, knowing.

"I don't know — I'm here to—" Alex can't get away from the child's eyes. Fear.

"I haven't seen him in three weeks. You here to tell me the son of a bitch is dead?"

Alex hands her the paperwork. "It's an eviction notice."

The child's eyes cut through her. "I'm sorry."

"You people are always sorry." The woman brushes the child away. "Get out of my goddamn hallway."

Slam.

.... *ten*

"Hey, Corine. Ten on number three." A man brushes past Alex, as if the car is going to flee.

Corine rings him up. The bangle bracelet queen. An older version of Alex. If she isn't careful.

"Hey, Alex. How's it goin'?"

"Hey." She leans on the counter. "Okay. Work's slow."

"Matt?"

Alex shrugs.

"He painting much?"

Another shrug. "I guess."

Corine opens a candy bar from the counter display and unwraps it. "Me and Eddie are going to San Diego for the weekend." She takes a bite. "He won it on the radio. I found out before he could take one of his buddies." She smiles proudly.

Alex looks out at the heat. "Wish I could get away."

Corine finishes the candy. Sticks the wrapper in the register. Listening to Alex.

"I mean. We."

.... *eleven*

The convertible sits outside the school. Alex watches the door. Drums restless fingers. Lays her head back.

Blows smoke at the sky.

The heat.

.... *twelve*

A stoplight turns green.

Alex stares through the windshield in a daze. Norma Jean watches her.

"It's green, Mama."

Black boots hesitate on the accelerator.

"Let's just drive, baby. Let's just drive and never stop." She looks at Norma Jean. Marilyn blowing on the dash.

"Okay." Norma Jean settles back.

Boots depress the pedal. The car pushes down the road.

"What about Daddy?" The question hangs.

Alex pulls Norma Jean's hair against her.

The lines disappear on the highway.

Hypnotic.

.... *thirteen*

Night.
Alex watches Norma Jean sleep.
Time lost.

.........*fourteen*

The Cadillac headlights pop on silently in the driveway. Wash across Matt's truck. Alex turns on the radio.

Matt listens to it in bed.

Stares at the glass angel he took from the box. Perfect, alone on the nightstand.

.........*fifteen*

Streetlights strobe against Marilyn.
On.
Off.
On.
The music blasts the night irreverently.
The bar finds the convertible.
The music pulls Alex inside.
The reckless stranger smiles.
His hands on her waist.
His knee between her thighs.
Her hands on his thighs.
Lips apart. Eyes closed. Head back. Breast sweaty.
The dance floor spins anonymity around her.

.... *sixteen*

The neon flashes a weary vacancy in the darkness.

Inside the room, the stranger tumbles with Alex in the sheets.

Grabbing.

Gasping.

"Never asked my name," he grunts at her.

She disappears under the sheets.

"Don't need to know."

.... *seventeen*

Pre-dawn. Alex pulls a t-shirt from the trunk of her convertible. Slips it on. Familiar routine.

Inside sprawled on twisted sheets the stranger lies unaware.

The wind whips Alex. And Marilyn.

Restless fingers drum the steering wheel.

Streetlights fade in a yawning sunrise.

A yellow stoplight burns red. The convertible squeals to a stop.

Punk lovers linger in the crosswalk. Hands all over each other.

Alex checks her reflection in the rearview. Wonders if he'll notice the bloodshot eyes.

Siren Red fingernails find the lipstick tube. Apply Siren Red to hesitant lips.

Alex blows herself a kiss.

Suddenly he's there. In the rearview. Kevin. Smiling. Rough and tumble. Snakeskin boots hover over motorcycle exhaust.

Steady, Alex hears her brain. Remember how to breathe.

Can't with your heart in your ears.

Black boots hover over the accelerator.

Too late. He has her on the driver's side. Leather sounds distracting. "Nice Caddy."

Alex guns the car. Willing the light green.

"Have a drink with me, Alex."

That smile. Shiver.

"That the best you can do after all this time, Kev?"

His lazy grin. "No."

The light flips to green.

Screech.

.........*eighteen*

Alex lights a cigarette in the kitchen. Hugs a cup of adrenaline.

Matt wanders past.

Coffee.

Cereal.

Silence.

"Didn't hear you come to bed."

Alex tugs at her t-shirt. "Fell asleep on the couch."

"Your father called." He watches her. Knowing. "Wants to visit."

Her hesitation.

His eyes.

Spoon against bowl. Clink. Clink.

Matt places his hand on the hood of the Cadillac. Pauses.

Still warm.

His chest tightens.

Reaches for the paper on the lawn. Headlines are the same. A wife shoots her husband. Didn't like the meatloaf.

.........nineteen

Alex rushes out of the plush office. Crashing sounds behind her.

"Son of a bitch!" The woman screams. "He's not getting the house!" Her high heel jabs a hole through the subpoena on the floor.

Alex stares at herself in the elevator doors.

Who is she?

A blow torch fires.

Matt sweats against the canvas.

Melting woman.

Burn.

.... *twenty*

Leather again.

"How's he treating you?" Kevin grins on the street.

"What do you want Kevin. Money?"

"He any fun? The kind of fun you like? Used to like?"

Alex glares at him. Even now those eyes. Mesmerizing.

"The reunion's real kick ass and all but I really don't have another goddamn thing to say to you." She tries to breathe normally.

Can't.

He moves closer.

"Can't fuck with destiny, Alex."

A slow sure smile.

"Thought you'd have that figured out by now."

She tears away from his eyes. Just get in the car. She can hear her brain screaming.

"I'm sure you're still the authority on what you can and cannot fuck." She adjusts the rearview.

Just breathe, Alex. Steady.

"But my destiny is sitting at school waiting for me to pick her up."

"American Pie taste like you thought?"

That voice. Her eyes close behind the sunglasses. Trouble.

Kevin guns off.

A breath escapes.

Matt yells from the kitchen. "Norma! Norma Jean!"

Sizzling pan. Singes himself. "Dammit. Norma!"

He marches into the living room to quiet the blaring monstrosity.

Norma Jean watches Carol Brady. Mom Perfecto. Buried in cookies and pepsi.

"Norma! Jean! You'll go deaf!"

She scowls.

"Don't have to yell, Daddy."

Cadillac silhouette against the sun.
Slender fingers.
Captive cigarette.
Mouth.
Eyes reflect burning clouds.

.... *twenty-one*

Matt and Norma eat.
Silence.
Clink.
"You mad, Daddy?"
"Yes."
"At me?"
"No."
The car engine outside. Matt stops. Norma too.
"Maybe it's Mama."
"Finish your dinner."
The door opens. Alex enters. Stops as they stare.
"You already ate. Good."
"Hi, Mama."
Matt burns. "Where you been?"
"Workin'."
They hold a stare. Knowing.
"You should have called, Mama. We worried."
Alex tousles Norma's hair.
"I should have. Sorry."
Matt pushes up. The chair slams. He storms out.
Norma's lip trembles. Alex cups her face. Eyes sorry.
"Don't worry. He's not mad at you, baby."
"I know. He's mad at you. For smoking."

.........twenty-two

Matt watches Alex undress by the bed.

He methodically eats the chocolate kiss. Rolls the wrapper. Tosses it in the corner.

Silence.

"Mike called."

Alex doesn't stop. "When?"

"Locked himself out of the office."

Alex shrugs. "He always locks himself out of the office."

Another wrapper arcs through the air. Rolls in the corner. Shiny.

"I asked where you were." Matt stares at her in the mirror. Knowing.

"Said you cut out early. Work being slow."

Siren Red nails click against the metal gun. She takes it from her belt. Lays it on the dresser.

"Matt. Don't."

Matt watches her fingers curve around the gun. Almost jealous.

"I don't want much, Alex."

"Everybody wants everything, Matt."

"No. I don't want anything. But you. Angel."

Alex bristles.

Matt watches her bare back. His eyes hold anger. Desperation. Sadness. "You're the only thing. Makes me happy."

Angry tears.

"You wanted this, Alex, you wanted this. Us. I don't understand."

She turns around. Brain imploding. "Look at me, Matt. I'm not your angel. This isn't. Happy."

"It's that job. That violence. It gets you upset. Makes you do things." Denial.

She stares. Eternally tired. "It's not the job, Matt."

Their eyes hold. A chasm between.

He turns over abruptly. "I'm tired now. I don't want to talk about this anymore." He pulls up the covers. Back to her.

"You can't keep putting this off. You have to face this. We need to separate Matt."

He closes his eyes. Unrelenting pain.

She stands over him. Guilty.

"God, if not for our sake. For Norma's."

She slips out.

He opens his eyes.

The gun.

Alex moves *Where The Wild Things Are* from Norma Jean's sleeping arms.

Slips into bed with her.

Holds her tight.

.... *twenty-three*

Siren fingernails fondle the edges of Matt's paintbrush. Unused.

Alex stares at the brush. Remembering why.

The Cadillac backs out of the drive.
Marilyn.
A corner rips in the breeze.

.... *twenty-four*

Fans beat the heavy air. Merciless.

Alex smokes at the window. Lost.

"Hold the fort down. I'm gone." Mike disappears.

Alex. Alone.

Sweat trickles. Shirt damp. Hands on temples.

Press out the heat.

If you can.

"How many sunsets he make you miss?"

Alex opens her eyes. There he is again.

He doesn't just watch. He consumes.

"Kevin, goddamnit. You're following me."

The leather smells good.

"You wanted me here."

Alex can't look away. "I didn't call you."

"Didn't have to."

More leather. Shiver.

"When you're with him. The bed feel empty?"

Alex can't find her voice. A whisper. "What do you want?"

Kevin moves closer. "I know what I want."

He sits her on the desk. Moves between her legs. "Do you know what you want?"

Try to breathe Alex.

Impossible.

"No." She barely gets it out.

Consuming kiss.

Neck back. Legs wrap.

"Forgot my keys." Mike is suddenly at the door.

"Mike…" Reality claws at Alex.

"Here they are. " He keeps going. He knows. "Like I said. Hold the fort down."

The lock clicks.

Her fists against his chest.

You can't do this again, Alex. Her brain screams.

You'll crash and burn.

Escape.

Now.

The Cadillac squeals from the curb.

A yellow stoplight burns red.

The Cadillac runs it.

Alex looks in the rearview.

Nothing.

She breathes.

Close.

Too close.

.... *twenty-five*

Desert road. Heat warps. Liquid car.
Alex inhales the wind.
Wishes the road was endless.
She checks the rearview again.
A dot on the horizon.
Black boots gun the accelerator.
Motorcycle wheels get closer.
Neck and neck they race.
Dangerous.
Fun.
The sun sinks.
Alex swerves at the motorcycle. Smiles.
The tires skid. The motorcycle spins off the road.
Kevin looks in his side mirror. A cut cheek.
He touches the blood.
Grins.
The horizon swallows the Cadillac.

Matt picks up Norma's toys. Puts them away carefully.
He watches her sleep.
Stares at the phone. Empty canvas leering.

Alex pulls up to a ridge. Dead halt.
She stands on the driver's seat. Screams at the blood red sky.

.... *twenty-six*

Alex sits against the tire. Lost in the shadows.

Full moon slides into the sky.

"You trying to kill me back there?" Kevin leans down. A hand on her thigh. "God I miss you."

Their eyes.

"Why is it I want to see you hanging from a goddamn freeway sign...and I still burn up all over when I get near you?" She knows there is no answer.

His hands under her shirt.

"We drew each other, Alex. You and me. That's all. Always comes back to that."

Her nails finger the buttons on his jeans. "I have this fantasy. About killing you." She touches the blood on his cheek.

Breast.

Mouth.

Back.

"How do I die?"

Bite. Groan.

"It's gruesome."

Skin. Sand. The sky.

.... *twenty-seven*

Sunrise glints off the chrome radio buttons.
A motorcycle roars.
Alex stirs in the backseat. Naked.
Slowly ascends to consciousness.
The motorcycle disappears down the road.
Alex watches. Tosses a bottle after it. "Bastard!"
The bottle shatters in the sand.
Alex looks at the convertible.
The tires are flat. Cut.
Marilyn is gone.

Out on the highway Kevin smiles.

.........*twenty-eight*

Black boots scuff along the pavement.

Siren fingers toss an empty cigarette pack on the deserted road.

Hot.

Alex stops. Looks at the empty expanse. Lights the last one.

A familiar Porsche pulls up. "Need a ride gorgeous?"

She takes another drag. Peers at Mike.

"What I need's another life."

Mike opens the door. "Get in line."

The blue sky rips past.

Restless Siren fingers. Hair blowing. Feet on the dash.

"So who's the guy?" Mike lights another cigarette. Passes it to her.

"Baggage. Unfinished business. A pain in the ass." She sucks on the cigarette.

Mike watches her legs. "A really good screw?"

Siren nails hang out the window. Feel the wind.

"Yeah. A really good screw."

A flashing stoplight. Stuck on yellow.

Clothes rain on the sidewalk. A man in the window screams to his lover on the street. Alex watches. Detached.

"I called a tow. Hey. Your tires were slashed."

Alex gets out of the Porsche. "Makes us even. You got a cigarette?"

He hands her the pack. "Your baggage?"

"Yeah." She watches the match ignite.

"Take a coupla days. On the house. Work out your thing."

"Thanks, Mike. I owe you."

"I know."

Alex watches him make an illegal hair brain u-turn. Just misses a truck. Obscenities scatter.

"Hey. What'd you do to him?" Mike yells from the car. An afterthought.

"Tried to run him off the road."

Mike contemplates. One complicated chick. He takes off.

Her smoke drifts aimlessly.

.... *twenty-nine*

Siren fingernails hesitate on the keys in the lock.

Finally turn them.

Inside the house the shades are drawn. A tomb.

"Matt?" Alex hears rustling in the shadows.

Then sees them.

Wrappers. All over. Thousands.

Matt stares at the TV. An old movie without sound. Black and white eyes.

He tosses another wrapper.

"Matt. Why are you sitting in the dark?"

He looks at her. "I was waiting for you to call. I didn't want to miss it."

Alex opens a blind. Lets in lines of light.

"Matt. I want to talk to you. About last night."

Matt presents her with his prize. "Look what I got. For us."

Alex stares numbly at the plane tickets.

"A second honeymoon. Just you and me. Angel."

Alex's brain implodes. "Don't call me that. I'm not."

"First one didn't count. We never left the studio." He takes her arm. She pulls away.

"Matt. No. We can't do this. I can't. Not another minute."

He isn't listening. "I packed. Corine's picking Norma up from school. We can leave now. Just go."

"Matt look at this. At me. It doesn't work. It only worked a little while at first. When I was numb. That's my fault. I wanted numb. But don't you see. I don't want numb anymore."

He doesn't see. Doesn't want to. "I can't watch you leave, Alex. I don't know what I'm supposed to do. I. Can't."

"It's time. To go. Let me. Go." She moves up the steps. He follows.

"No." He pulls at her. "You can't. I can't do this. Without you."

She grabs her suitcase. Throws things in. No order.

"Don't you want to know where I was last night? Who I was with? Can't you for once at least get mad, fight, something?"

Siren nails grab the handle. She spins down the steps.

"Whatever you want me to do. I'll do. Anything. Just. Tell me." He follows.

"We can talk about Norma Jean. Later." Alex opens the door. "I need to think right now. Leave her with Corine."

She can't stand the pain in his eyes.

"You're tired. We can fix it. We can talk. Later." He fights the tears.

Alex can't stand it. "You and your goddamn picket fence and your happy endings and your goddamn guilt…"

Matt sinks to the steps.

"I'm sorry for trying to make this fit. I thought. I could be somebody else. I wish…" Alex watches the sunshine outside. The freedom. "Well. It's a little late for wishes now."

"I love you, Allie."

She plunges into the light.

The door closes. Encasing him in darkness.

The wedding painting haunting in the shadows.

.... *thirty*

"'Please stay. Don't go. We'll eat you up we love you so. And Max said No!'" Alex reads. Snuggled in billows of fabric with Norma Jean.

Norma stares at The Wild Things' fangs. Into their eyes.

Alex holds her face.

"I love you, baby. You are. Real special. I don't ever want you to let anybody else tell you different."

The light sparkles on the snow globes and glass crystals at Corine's.

"Why'd you stop, Mama?"

"Listen to me, Norma Jean."

"What about Max? What about The Wild Things?"

"Baby, this is important."

Light speckles dance over them.

"Baby, I'm going to go away for a few days. You're going to stay here with Corine. Is that okay with you?"

Norma isn't sure. "Where are you going?"

"Somewhere I can think."

"About what?"

"Listen, baby, when I get back we'll talk about it. Right now I don't know how to explain it all to you."

"Is Daddy mad at me?"

"No, baby. He's not mad."

Alex's eyes spill. Looking at the miniature version of herself. Her soul. So much ahead to love. To fight.

"I'm. Sorry. For all of this, baby. I'll make it up to you. Somehow. I'll figure it all out. I promise."

Norma touches Alex's face gently. Her innocent eyes hold all the trust in the world. "Don't cry, Mama. It'll be okay."

She turns the page for Alex. "Read about how he sails back to his room and supper's still hot."

Cinderella and Prince Charming watch from inside their snow dome trapping.

The cigarette glow on the porch step lights up Corine's face.

"What did he do?"

Alex sighs at the darkness. "Nothing."

"So why do you have to leave?"

"I can't stand 'nothing' anymore."

"What about that baby in there?" Corine takes a deep drag. "What about that?"

"I know. I swear I feel like Sibyl. All torn up. Matt pulls me this way. Norma Jean pulls me that way. And all the rest just keeps bubblin' up inside. Pulling me. I don't know. Somewhere else."

"Life just isn't picture perfect like a catalogue, Alex. Eddie pops me now and then. So what? He keeps me warm at night. He's someone to talk to in the morning. Besides, I burn his dinner when he gets rough. It all evens out." Candid reality.

Alex looks at Corine. You're not so far from that kind of future, Alex. If you're not careful. She shivers in the warm night air. "I tried. I really tried."

The smoke trails up to the stars.

The wind chimes catch the hot air sweetly.

Corine smiles.

"He still hasn't found that bowling bag I threw out last week."

.........*thirty-one*

A stoplight burns red.

The convertible idles.

Black boots hover on the accelerator. Siren nails tap the steering wheel.

The bar across the street drips neon into the night.

Kevin's motorcycle sits in the lot.

Alex smiles.

"Over there, hon." Alex legs walk beside the big tattooed man as he pushes the motorcycle. Watching her thighs.

"Sure thing, sweetheart. How about a drink?"

Alex flicks the cigarette into a puddle of grease.

"I'll take a rain check."

The motorcycle sits perfectly in the fountain. The angel spouting water over it. Wings reaching for the night.

Kevin runs toward it. "Fuck!"

Jumps in. "Son of a bitch!"

He wrestles to drag it out.

Sits. Drenched.

Stares.

Laughs at the moon.

.... *thirty-two*

The motel television plays "Bus Stop".

Alex half-watches the images. Curled on the bed. Phone cradled to her ear. A twelve year old's memories. "Hi, Mama."

Marilyn fills the screen.

"No. Everything's fine. I just wanted to hear your voice...No...don't put Daddy on."

Siren nails twist the cord.

"Hi, Daddy. No everything's fine. Yes. He's fine. Everything's. Fine."

Marilyn cries.

Alex. Filled with doubt. "Yeah. I'm taking real good care of him. Both of them. No, she's asleep. I'll tell him you said hey. Yeah. I know. He's a 'winner'. Yes. I'm still your. Baby doll."

She takes a swig of beer to wash down the words.

"You don't sound far away either."

Guilt. The lies.

"Bye, Daddy."

Marilyn. Mesmerizing pain.

"No, Mama. Yes, I still carry it. It's a gun for god sakes. Of course it's loaded. Mama, I don't want to fight about my job. Just. Mama. I'm grown. No...Mama, I gotta go. No...everything's. Fine. Really."

She hangs up. Lays her head down.

Marilyn's eyes flicker on the tube.

The pool lights illuminate the water. Alex cuts through the soothing liquid. No sound. No sorrow. No today. No yesterday.

A black cowboy boot floats past her to the bottom.

She dives for the boot. Her favorite pair.

Breaks through the top. Furious.

"Hey!" She throws the boot at Kevin. He smiles lazily. Poolside. "Son of a bitch!"

He ducks the boot. "Thanks for the car wash. Wanna go dancing?"

"Fuck you."

"Hey, we're even now. Like always, Alex."

"We were even when I watered your bike."

"So think of something. To do." He watches the water lick at her breasts. He slips in. Walks towards her. "Something good."

"Fuck you."

"You said that already."

Alex runs a hand through wet hair. He watches her mouth. Wet. "I'm tired of this. Kevin."

"No you're not. You love it."

She trembles.

"You need it. Like me. You can't breathe without it. Not knowing."

He pushes her onto the steps. The water laps her legs. Her fingers clutch the cement. Breathe Alex. Remember how. Just. Breathe.

He kneels between her legs. "You're a hurricane, sweetheart. Not fucking Mrs. Right." He kisses her thigh.

She locks her legs around his neck.

Squeeze.

Choke.

Dunk.

Thrash.

Again.

Struggle.

Finally let go.

Kevin gasps for air. "Jesus Christ!"

"They were my favorite boots." A long wet kiss. "So. Dancing?"

She climbs out of the pool.

Kevin watches her.

Fuck.

The blowtorch melts the canvas.

Savage.

Sputters out. Suddenly.

"Allie, that you?" Matt listens for the door.

His eyes.

Hope.

Anguish.

.... *thirty-three*

Mass of bodies. Tangled. Music.
Kevin and Alex pumping in the epicenter.
Breathless.
Bodies made for each other.
They weave to a table.

A dozen empty glasses. They laugh uncontrollably. Try to look at each other sober.

Can't.

Burst.

Stares.

Late. Silence. Confession hour.

Siren fingers caress the cigarette. "God. It's been too damn long since we did this."

"About your ball and chain..."

Alex cuts him a dark look. "No."

Kevin grins. "Come on. Let's have some fun with him."

"He's not in this, Kevin."

Kevin's eyes go black. Smile fades. "He's not just gonna let you walk away, sweetheart."

"I already have."

Kevin drinks. "He's still got your kid."

That scares her. He knows it.

Her eyes. "Corine's keeping her. For now. But he'll let me. Take her."

Kevin leans close. "I wouldn't."

Alex holds his stare. "I know."

.... *thirty-four*

The convertible races at breakneck speed.

Kevin watches Alex stand.

Hold on. Feel the wind.

A whoop.

The tires turn sharply. Barrel off the road.

Alex lurches forward. Screams. "Kevin!"

Rocky. Bumpy.

"Yes? Dear?"

"What are you doing? Where does this go?"

Wild eyes. Grin. "Got me."

The tires spin faster. The headlight beams bob dangerously.

Suddenly the cliff is on them. Almost past them.

Alex screams.

Kevin skids. Laughing.

The convertible slides to the edge.

Almost doesn't stop.

Alex's forehead hits the dash.

Blood.

The waves pound below.

Kevin bolts out. Leans too far. Screams at the sea. "Alex! Come on! Let's swim!"

"No." Dizzy.

He pulls her out of the car. Drags her to the edge. Undresses her.

"My head hurts." Fuzzy.

"And your lungs are poppin' and your heart's trippin'. While the rest of the world's goin' numb on fuckin' Nytol."

His eyes. On fire.

The blood on her hands.

She touches it.

Fear.

Alex's silhouette in the motel window. Straddling him. Riding hard.

His hands pull the silk scarf tight on her neck.

She arches. Gasping for air.

Goes limp.

Silk trails loosely against nipple.

She pants against his chest.

Pleasure.

Pain.

A bucket of soapy water inside the trashed studio. Matt calmly polishes the same spot on the studio floor.

Over and over.

Cinderella.

The painting watches him in the background.

The glass angel's wings lay in a ruined rage beside him.

Matt touches the glass.

Exhausted.

Tears.

Later. Alex stares at Kevin sprawled. Asleep.
Siren fingernails dig for a cigarette.
Start to light the match. Tremble.
Can't.
Head in hands. Crash and burn, Alex.
Crash and burn.

.... *thirty-five*

The motel neon buzzes off in the sunrise.

Kevin plays with the gun chamber.

Click. Click.

Alex sleeps. Oblivious to dawn.

A leggy dancer shimmies across the parking lot. Next to nothing top. Transparent chiffon skirt.

Opens the wrong door. "Oh. Sorry."

Kevin points the gun at the dancer.

She freezes.

Pulls the trigger.

Click.

She screams. Alex bolts up. Stares at the dancer. Confused.

Kevin grins. "Just kidding. Lighten up."

"Bastard." She slams the door.

The window's blinding light cuts at Alex wickedly. Head like concrete. "Who was that?"

"One skinny chick with absolutely no sense of humor." He opens the chamber. "He bring you breakfast in bed?" He puts a hand on her breast.

She holds her head. "I'm taking about three thousand aspirin. And then I'm packing."

"I already packed. Let's drive down to Mexico."

Alex tries to get up. "I'm not going to Mexico. I can't leave Norma any longer. I've gotta go back."

She manages to get in the shower.

Inside the chamber. One lone bullet.

Alex steps through the steam. Reaches for a towel.
Sees the red scrawl on the mirror.
'CAN'T FUCK WITH DESTINY'.
She hears the convertible roar. "Kevin?"

She runs outside. Kevin pulls out in the convertible. Her suitcase in the back. He turns on the radio. Waving. Laughing at her reflection in the rearview.

"Vaya con deee-asss, baby."

The dancer stands in the doorway in a dowdy bathrobe. Watching too. Alex turns.

"He took everything."

"They usually do."

Alex pulls at her wedding ring. "Look, I'll trade you."

The dancer stares at the ring. "Now what the hell am I gonna do with that?"

"I don't have anything else."

"That's your whole problem sister."

.... *thirty-six*

The highway lines disappear. Hypnotic.

The stoplight turns red.

The truck cab pulls up. Stops.

Alex climbs out. The dancer's costume. White dress. White heels.

"Hey. Thanks."

The truck honks and rattles off.

Alex's dress blows up over the grate.

Just like Marilyn.

.... *thirty-seven*

The fans beat the air thickly. Alex leans in Mike's door.

"I feel like a hooker."

Mike looks up at her. "You look like one. I like it."

Alex lights a cigarette. Takes a deep drag. "He took my car. My clothes. Left me at the hotel. I had to buy this off a dancer. Bastard."

She inspects a run. Mike watches her fingers trace it.

"Guess that answers my question about your weekend."

"Can I borrow your car?"

Mike tosses her the keys. "I keep some fresh shirts in the trunk. For. You know."

Alex nods. "Yeah. Me too."

"Help yourself. You gonna be okay?"

Alex closes her eyes against the heat. "Who? Daddy's baby doll? Matt's angel? Kevin's hurricane? Norma's Mama?"

Mike shrugs. "Hey. I'm sittin' here with no answers."

He watches her blow smoke in tiny rings. "Which one's Alex?"

"I don't know. What if they're all me. All at once."

Another shrug. "Couldn't tell you. I'm one dimensional. It's less of a hassle."

She stares at the keys. Vulnerable. "Hey. Thanks. Guess I owe you. Again."

"Get outta here in that thing. Before I ask you to pay up."

Alex wafts out.

Mike fantasizes.

Tantalizing chiffon.

.... *thirty-eight*

White high heels stop at Matt's truck.

Alex stares up at the house.

Everything in its place.

Inside she passes the glass angel. Fingers its broken wing. Pauses. Walls closing in.

"Matt?"

No answer.

She climbs to the bedroom. Dark. Closed up.

Matt between the sheets. Curled up. Unmoving. "Matt."

"Allie."

She opens the windows. Back to him.

"I thought. I dreamed it. You. Leaving."

She bristles. "It wasn't a dream."

The sunlight hits the candy wrappers on the floor. "How long since you ate real food?" She turns around.

His face is drenched in sweat. His eyes glazed.

She rushes to him. "Matt!"

"I know it wasn't a dream. I kept waking up. And you were gone. And I didn't want. To be alive."

Suddenly Alex sees the soup bowl. She picks it up. Smells it. "What did you put in the soup, Matt?"

His eyes close. He drifts. "I'm just so tired. Let me sleep. For a minute."

Alex pulls at him. Frantic. "Matt, I want you to try and sit up. Come on." She tries to drag him up. He is too big for her.

"Come on. Help me, baby. We've gotta get you to the doctor."

He sags into her. “I didn’t think you were coming back. Don’t leave me again. Like that.”

Alex swims in guilt.

.... *thirty-nine*

Alex leans against the hospital corridor wall. Drops another butt in the ashtray.

Mike appears. "What's the word?"

"He tried to poison himself. But he didn't take enough to. Die."

"Just enough to get your attention."

"Which he got." She tosses Mike his keys. "I have the truck. Thanks."

"Need anything?"

She inhales. Nods no.

"Where you staying?"

"There." She puts the cigarette out.

"How long?"

She shrugs. " 'Til it's over. I guess."

Mike puts an arm around her. "If you need anything."

She touches his arm. Grateful. "Yeah. I know."

The tangled web.

.........*forty*

The sunset burns the expanse of sky.

Alex leans against the truck.

Weary.

The more she tries to breathe...the more she seems to smother.

No way out.

.........forty-one

The truck pulls into the drive. Alex sucks in her breath.

The convertible is parked in the driveway.

She clicks the headlights off. Uneasy.

Inside the door she hesitates. Calls out in the dark.

"Kevin?"

Nothing.

Room to room.

Shadows.

Breath short.

"Kevin. Dammit. If you're here."

Up the stairs. Slowly.

Darkness. Creaking somewhere.

Wedding picture gruesome in the shadows.

Her heels crunch the shiny wrappers strewn around.

Alex pauses by the bed. The phone rings beside her.

She jumps. Heart pounding. "God."

Another ring. "Hello? Oh. Corine."

Relief.

Behind her in the shadows. Kevin. Eyes on fire.

"I just can't deal with it all tonight. I don't know what to say to her. About Matt. About anything."

Kevin watches. Not moving.

"Look. Would you mind watching her another night? And I'll get her in the morning. Don't tell her I'm back yet."

Kevin sees. Her nylon run.

"Corine. All I did was try to be honest. Leave. This isn't. I didn't cause this."

Corine cooks at the stove. A black eye. Billowing smoke. "You left the man, Alex. And took his child. You tore up his life." She hangs up the phone. Yells. "Dinner's ready."

Black goo.

Alex hangs up. Behind her. No Kevin.

She slips in bed. Reaches for the remote.

Pauses at the picture of her Dad. Looming over her and Matt at the wedding table. Hand on each shoulder. Pushing them together for the picture.

Matt looking at her. Her looking at her Dad.

Approval.

A hand grabs her wrist. Her scream jerks her out of reverie.

Kevin. The gun. "I say let's end the day with a bang."

Alex watches him cock it. "No more games, Kev."

He pushes it toward her. "It'll be fun."

"No."

"Me first." He points it at himself.

"Kevin. Don't."

Her eyes.

Mouth.

Sweat.

"Don't worry. There's only one bullet. That's what makes it fun, Alex."

He grins. Pulls the trigger.

Alex lunges. "No!"

Click. He shrugs. "Your turn." He cocks the gun again.

"Pretty please?" Points it at her.

Sweat.

"Kevin. Stop." She whispers a plea.

"Is your heart pounding in your ears yet, Alex?"

Siren fingernails tremble. Clutch at the covers.

"Don't you feel it, Alex? The rush?"

He reaches out to feel a tear.

"Kevin. Please."

He pulls the trigger. She screams.

Click. He grins. "You're losing your nerve, Alex. You're out of practice."

She throws a pillow at him. "Son of a bitch!"

He shoots it mid-air.

The pillow explodes.

Feathers.

Alex splashes her face in the sink. Trying to stop shaking.

"Just come with me. We can go to Carlita's motel. Like always."

Alex leans her forehead on the sink. Nauseous. "I was bored. But this. I can't keep up, Kev. You have to go."

He rubs her waist with his hands. Behind her. "We were so good in Mexico."

"I have to stay here. Matt. Needs me here. I have to tell Norma Jean."

He kisses her neck. She closes her eyes. Fighting sensation.

He grins. Lazy. "You'll change your mind. Eventually. Lotta nights to fill."

He turns on the TV.

Marilyn again.

Slams the door on his way out.

Alex sinks to the floor.

Sobs.

.........*forty-two*

Alex lies outstretched on the tiles. Exhausted sleep.

The bell rings.

Again.

Again.

Alex opens her eyes. Hears it.

Makes her way downstairs. Mike is on the doorstep. She peers at him. Numb. "Mike."

"Just checking on you."

"You could have called."

"Yeah. I could have." He walks inside.

"Want a drink?" She rubs her eyes.

"No. But you look like you could use one."

She begins to tremble. Covers her face. Shaking. "I just want to get him out of my system."

Mike leads her to the couch. Sits her down. "Looks like he's one of those lifetime viruses." He fixes a drink. "I've found this to be the best cure for that."

Alex downs it in one gulp.

Mike stares at a portrait of her. A body without a face. Curves with no identity. "Did you eat?"

Candles burn low. Empty plates. Siren fingernails play with silverware. "My problem is I always liked it. Wondering if we were going to go too far. It made the sex incredible. It made my life a nightmare. It was a constant high. I got too dizzy. So I left him. Went looking for a big dose of normal."

Mike pours more liquid. "Doesn't exist."

She sighs. "That was five years ago. Right before Matt. And his soft words and his easy way. Right before Norma Jean was born."

She lights a cigarette. "And there hasn't been a day I haven't expected him to show up in the driveway. Even hoped he would."

Mike takes a cigarette from her pack. "And now that he has?"

She stares past the smoke. "I'm terrified he won't leave. What's funny is, I couldn't breathe being in the middle of something exciting all the time. And I can't breathe in the middle of all this. Predictability."

Mike watches her lips. Her eyes. Vulnerable looks good on her. "There are all kinds of asphyxiation: Obsession. Depression. Oppression. Guilt. Most of 'em are legal."

He stacks the dishes. Rises.

"Thanks. For dinner." She smiles. Grateful.

"Hey. A new angle on the life thing I'm useless. Can openers I know."

He runs water. Stares at her reflection in the window.

The candles smoke.
Alex sleeps. Legs across Mike's lap.
He sips a drink. Watches her sleep.
She moves, vulnerably, snuggles close. Still asleep.
He leans close.
Her lips so soft.
Almost.
Doesn't.

.........*forty-three*

The hospital television emits June Cleaver. Happy in the kitchen.

Alex kisses Matt's forehead. Maternal.

"Allie."

"How do you feel?"

"Are you back? To stay?"

"I don't think we should talk about that right now."

June makes more cookies. Alex sits. Watching.

"You really scared me, Matt."

"I got so depressed last night. After your friend stopped by." Apologetic eyes. "I didn't mean..."

Alex whips around. "Friend?"

Matt nods. "Kevin."

Siren fingernails grip the blanket.

"What did he. Do."

Matt watches June iron. "Said he'd run into you and you wanted me to know you were okay."

Fingernails relax.

Matt stares at her sadly. "I was thinking about the first time you modeled for me."

She smiles. Sad too. "For rent money."

"I wish I knew what you wanted. So I could do it, Alex."

His eyes well with frustration.

"I don't want you to do anything else for me. Except get better."

Guilt.

.... *forty-four*

The stoplight turns green.

Red.

The convertible idles.

A wall plastered with bills stretches away from Alex. A dozen Marilyn headshots stare back at her. Laughing.

But the artist added a tear.

.........*forty-five*

Corine opens the door. Yells off to Eddie. "I have no idea where your damn tool set is."

She smiles at Alex. "Hey there."

"Hey. Guess I have to explain this to Norma Jean. I don't know what to say."

Confusion. "What do you mean? Norma's gone."

"What?"

"Your friend came to get her."

Dizzy. "Friend?"

"Kevin. I'd take him home in a heartbeat."

Alex is already running toward the car. "Kevin? You let him take her?"

Corine. Unconcerned. "Didn't you give him my address?"

Alex guns the motor. "Where were they going?"

"He said you knew where you were supposed to meet him. Hey. Where you off to? And what's with him? Where'd you meet him?"

Alex spins off.

"And why didn't you introduce me?"

Dust.

Kevin's motorcycle does a wheelie.

Norma Jean holds on. Screaming.

Eyes laughing. Hair whipping wildly.

The rush.

.... *forty-six*

The convertible passes cars. Too tight.
Siren fingers on the steering wheel.
A nervous cigarette.
The diner. A mirage in the sweltering heat.
Alex pulls up. Leans in the phone booth.
A deep drag.
She dials Mike.
Empty ringing.
She hangs up. Dials him at home.
Nothing.
She leans against the phone. Exhausted.
You can't lose the game, Alex. Not this time.
Not this one.

.... *forty-seven*

The battered road sign to Mexico is barely visible. Tired horizon almost spent.

Alex pulls off the road. Gets out. Engine running.

She pulls the magnetic metal gun case from under the wheel well. Opens it. Reaches into the glove compartment for her gun.

Gasps.

Empty.

"Oh, god." Kevin's roulette flashes through her mind.

His grin.

She slams the car door. Head against the steering wheel.

"Oh, baby. I'm sorry. I'm so sorry."

She turns on the lights.

Wipes her eyes.

Steel.

No turning back.

The convertible rips toward the border.

The empty gun case still in the dirt.

.... *forty-eight*

The convertible pulls into Carlita's motel.

Headlight beams cut across Kevin's motorcycle.

Alex turns off the engine. Reaches for the lights.

A little girl prostitute passes in the light. Catches Alex's eye.

The ancient man with her pushes her along.

Alex kills the lights.

.... *forty-nine*

Kevin lies on the bed. Boots on. Jeans.

Bare chest.

Eyes flutter. Inebriated dreams.

Empty beer bottles litter the bed. The night table.

The TV blares "How To Marry A Millionaire."

Marilyn in Spanish.

Siren fingernails wrap around the gun silently.

A bottle flies through the air. Hits the headboard by Kevin's ear. He bolts up.

A hungover grin. "Told you you'd change your mind."

Alex isn't playing. "Where is she?"

"At Grandma's. Dear."

Alex wavers. Surprised. "Why? What?"

"Because it's what you really want. You just won't admit it."

"No." Alex finds her voice. "I love her."

"Face it, Alex. You know it. I know it. You weren't cut out to go to Mother Daughter Girl Scout banquets."

His power. Cutting to her doubt.

He reaches for her breasts. "Hey. World doesn't need any more Girl Scouts."

Her eyes glint. Finding the will. "Remember my fantasy?"

She climbs on top of him.

"I like it so far." Kevin watches. Curious pleasure.

She kisses his neck.

Face to face. Tears stream.

He licks them off.

The gun inches down to his chest. Feather light.

His breath quickens.

Alex kisses his lips. Teasing.

The gun trails down to his zipper.

His eyes close.

Groan.

Siren fingernails cock the gun.

Kevin's eyes open wide at the click. Suddenly. Terror.

Alex's eyes. Hard. "Can you feel the rush yet, Kevin? Isn't this. Fun." She bites his lip.

He tastes the blood. Nervous.

"Don't fight it, Alex. Give in. Stay. You're free. You are not what they think. I know."

Her hands tremble.

His eyes. For the first time. Real fear. He goes for her doubt again. "We drew each other."

His hand moves toward hers. The gun.

She searches his face. Wavering. Lost. "Destiny?"

He strokes a breast. "This is the only time you feel alive. You know that."

Try to breathe Alex. Try.

Can't.

Closes her eyes. Confusion. "But. Norma."

Kevin's hand slips over the gun. "You're tired of the responsibility."

Alex's eyes. Tears. Doubt. "Yes."

He slips her hands from the gun. Rolls her beneath him. Crushing her movement. "You hate Matt for being so easy."

Whisper. "Yes."

Soothing kiss. "You hate his pathetic attempt to kill himself."

Inaudible. “Yes.”

He traces a lip. “Let the rest of the world choke down their feelings over their Corn Flakes. You. You want more. You always have.”

His eyes. On fire. “Our version of reality’s better. It’s right here, Alex. Take it.”

His hands beneath her underwear.

His mouth.

Her gasp.

Siren nails dig into the headboard.

Marilyn.

.... *fifty*

Two parents fight in the diner. A little boy sits between. Crying.

Alex watches the child.

Kevin eats. Buried in newspaper headlines. "Some guy blew his wife's head off. Went to her office. Blam. Jesus, he should have just left. Or had an affair."

The parents scream louder. The man knocks his plate out of the way and walks off. The woman runs after. Hitting him. Jostles Alex as she passes.

Coffee spills on her shirt. "Oh. Great. I don't have another shirt. Clean."

She watches the woman drag the child past.

His eyes. So full of the violence.

Alex scoots out. "I'll borrow one of yours."

Kevin ignores her. Buried in someone else's misery. "Lady cut her fiancee up night before the wedding. Jesus. World's a fucking mess anymore."

Alex watches the little boy disappear into a car in the parking lot. Still crying.

She finds Kevin's duffel bag near the phone in the room. She dials Mike. Opening the bag. Digging for a t-shirt. "Mike?"

In his office, Mike looks out the window. Worried. "Alex, where the hell are you? I called..."

"Mexico."

She pulls out a photo of Kevin. With her. Years ago in Mexico. She stares at it.

"What are you doing down there?"

"Long story."

"Oh." Mike knows not to ask.

"I just wanted to tell you I won't be at work. Yet. Will you check on Matt for me?"

"Already have. They've put him on the psych ward. Which he is not happy about. Keeps denying the suicide attempt."

"God. I just wish. He'd let go."

"He's pretty adamant. Says he felt fine. Until he ate. He's asking about you."

"I'll be back."

Mike turns from the window. "Why don't I believe you?"

"Bye, Mike."

Mike stares at the phone a beat. Grabs his coat. Leaves.

Alex puts the picture back in the duffel bag.

Sees a pill bottle next to it.

The label. Poison.

Alex sinks to the bed. Dizzy. Kevin at Matt's. The soup.

She dials Mike again.

Tremble. "Oh, god. Mike. Pick up. Please."

No answer.

Kevin's shadow suddenly blocks the sunlight in the door frame.

Siren fingers conceal the bottle. Push it under the pillow.

Kevin stares evenly. "Thought you'd run off and left me."

"Now why would I do that, baby?" She takes off her shirt.

Kevin closes the door.

Matt pounds the walls of the little white room. Screams at the door. "Listen to me! Listen to me!"

He slides down the wall. "Listen to me..."

His eyes.

Something off.

Alex pants raggedly on the floor.

Sweat.

Kevin zips his pants. "I'm bored. Let's find a cantina."

Alex heads for the bathroom. "I gotta rinse off. Give me a few minutes."

Kevin lounges on the bed. Watches her nude body disappear into the bathroom. Flips on the TV.

Alex closes the bathroom door. Grips the sink. Tries not to vomit.

She stares at herself.

Terror.

Turns on the shower. Grabs a towel.

Climbs out the window.

Her bare feet pad the dirt.

Siren fingernails disconnect Kevin's brakeline.

Alex gets in the convertible.

Sees the lipstick on the dash.

She has to.

She climbs out. Scrawls on Kevin's rearview.

Climbs back in.

Stares at the ignition. "Shit."

She leans under to jump start it. Rusty.

Kevin digs for a clean shirt. Sees the poison bottle gone.

He hears the convertible start.

Bolts out of the room. "Alex!"

Alex drives. Wind whipping bare skin.

Goose bumps on her thighs.

Kevin mounts the motorcycle.

FUCK DESTINY on the rearview. His eyes snap. He screams again. A wounded animal. "ALEX!!!"

The convertible goes faster.

Alex watches him in the rearview. Gaining.

He screams in the wind.

She can't hear him.

Neck and neck.

They race.

Suddenly the ravine opens its jaw.

Alex presses the brake. Wheels skid short of the drop.

Kevin tries his brakes.

Nothing.

He shoots past her.

Over the edge.

"Alex!" Their eyes hold as he drops into the darkness.

Siren fingernails grip the steering wheel.

Knuckles white.

Engine running. "Oh shit. Oh shit."

Finally Alex gets out. Looks over the ravine.

Snakeskin boots tangled grotesquely in the dirt.

Blood.

Crushed chrome.

Alex stands at the edge. Sucks in the air.

Try to breathe, Alex. Try.

Can't.

.... *fifty-one*

Alex shivers in the phone booth. Struggling into a dress snatched from a clothesline.

"Mike. I don't have time to explain. Get Norma Jean for me and meet me at the Motel 6 outside of town. I'll be there as soon as I can. She's at my parent's — number's — oh fuck, it's listed. Farini. Alexander."

Mike listens in bed. Alone. "You're a junior too? Explains a lot."

Whisper. "Oh God."

"Alex, I'll come get you. You sound bad. What happened?" Her voice tears a hole in him.

"Things have been. Down hill. Ever since I lost Marilyn."

"What?"

"Nothing."

"Corine can get Norma. Tell me where you are."

"Don't try to be a knight at this late date, baby. Just get Norma Jean. Promise."

"I promise." He hangs up. Sits in the dark.

Alex sighs.

.... *fifty-two*

The night blows past.

Siren fingernails on the steering wheel.

Music too loud.

Alex approaches the border. Slows.

Sandwiched between cars.

Reaches for a cigarette. Restless.

Empty pack.

Opens the glove compartment.

"Shit." The gun is now inside.

The car in front of her moves up. Alex watches border patrol search the trunk.

Sweat.

"You and your goddamn games." She can almost hear his grin.

She slips the gun beneath the seat.

Pulls up.

Border patrol stares at her sternly.

"What happened to your shoes? Have to leave someplace in a hurry?"

"I like to drive barefoot. Officer." She manages a slow smile.

"Could you step out of the car, please?"

Alex moistens her lips. Breathe Alex. Breathe. "I'd be happy to. Officer."

She climbs out of the convertible.

He eyes her chest. "Can I see your registration?"

"Sure thing." She reaches across the seat for the paperwork from the glove compartment. The officer watches her ass. Thighs stretching.

He smiles at the other officer. "Could I have the key to the trunk, please?" Control.

Alex's heart. Racing. Don't notice the keys gone. "Doesn't lock."

He pops the trunk open. Alex watches. Better not have left any more surprises. Bastard.

The officer stands. Staring inside.

Alex tries to swallow. Throat thick.

He finally slams the trunk. Ready to intimidate the next car. "Okay." He pats the trunk.

Alex smiles. Shaky. "Have a nice evening, officer."

Her heel against the gun.

"You too, ma'm." He leers.

A gold cap.

.... *fifty-three*

Alex throws down a carton of Marlboro's in front of the punk clerk. Already open. Already smoking one.

"Rough night?" He rings her up.

"Just a hopeless chain smoker."

She sees the circular rack of Marilyn postcards next to the register.

Marilyn's eyes.

She scuffs outside. Hugs herself. Closes her eyes.

Tries not to see Kevin. Lying there.

Blows a huge cloud of smoke at the sky.

Slaps a Marilyn postcard on the dash.

Crash and burn, Alex.

Crash and burn.

Rear lights on.

Engine.

.... *fifty-four*

The Motel 6 sign sears the night.

Alex pulls in beside Mike's Porsche. Rests her head.

Finally here.

Inside, Mike puts a finger to his lips.

Norma Jean curled asleep in the bed.

Mike looks at the skimpy dress. Bare feet. "I won't ask. You okay?"

Alex pushes past him to Norma. Sinks by the bed. "It's okay now. Everything's okay."

"You sure?"

Alex's eyes fill at the sight of her little woman. She touches Norma's forehead. Pulls the cover up gently. "He's gone. He won't be back."

She looks at Mike. Grateful. Molds herself against him in a hug.

Mike tries to recover.

"Thanks, Mike."

"I know. You owe me."

"I do." Alex smiles into his eyes.

His lips hesitate. Then cover hers.

His hands move over her hips. She starts to give in. Familiar routine.

They move into the bathroom.

Press against the wall.

Rough.

Suddenly Alex pushes him away. Realization. Blinding her.

She stares at him a beat.

He watches her. Confused.

"Gratitude." Siren fingernails rebutton her dress. Determined. "Like you said. It's just another way to suffocate."

His eyes flash. Angry.

"I'm trying to remember that, Mike."

He grabs his keys.

"You don't have to go."

He's out the door. "Yeah. I do."

The Porsche guns out. Alex watches from the door.

Closes it.

In the lamplight Norma Jean looks like an angel.

.... *fifty-five*

Angry sun. Intense.

The convertible sits outside the house. Alex doesn't pull it into the driveway.

She looks at the porch. Shutting out the twelve year old's memories.

Her father and mother at the door. Watching. Stern.

"Norma Jean!" He yells for her.

Norma bolts out of the house, racing towards Alex. The car.

He stops her. Smiles down. "This is for grampa's baby doll." The package slips into her tiny arms.

Alex sucks on a cigarette. Watching him. Empty.

Norma smiles. "Love you, Grampa." She bolts off.

"You be good now." His eyes follow her. To Alex. Smile fading.

The convertible cruises through the desert.

Norma Jean rips into the package. Delight.

"It's a book! Who's that girl?"

Alex cuts a look at the book. Sees the girl. Irritation. "Sleeping Beauty."

"Why is she sleeping?"

"She's waiting for this prince. To come wake her up."

Norma Jean considers this. "She shouldn't wait. She should play."

Alex smiles. "Yes. She should."

Alex takes the book and throws it out the window.

Norma Jean watches it flutter through the air.

"Say good bye, Beauty."

They giggle. Together. "GOOD-BYE, BEAUTY!!!"

They drive silently.

Alex finds the words. "I want you to know something, baby. Things are going to be messy for awhile. But your Daddy and I love you. And everything's gonna be fine."

"Why's it going to be messy, Mama?"

Alex watches the book pages swirling in the rearview. "It's just how life gets sometimes. That's all."

.... *fifty-six*

A stoplight. Stuck on yellow.
Alex drops Norma Jean at school.
A little girl kisses a little boy.
He wipes it off.

.... *fifty-seven*

Alex walks into the courthouse.
Thinks she sees Kevin on the motorcycle across the street.
A truck passes.
Her heart pounds.
She looks again.
Nothing's there.
Don't lose it, Alex.
Don't crack now.

"How you feel?" Mike is cool. Alex feels the edge between them.

"I don't know."

"You going to tell me what happened down there in Mexico?"

"No. It's over. No point talking about it."

Mike watches her legs. Irritated. "This mean you're back to work?"

Alex paces. "I can't. Handle. I mean. Right now. Look. Will you help Matt? Get out of this psych thing? I want to...Get on with things."

Mike stares. Hard. "I'll go see him this afternoon."

Alex leans across the desk and kisses his cheek. "Thanks, Mike. You're a good friend. I need. A good friend. Right now."

She walks out.
Doesn't see him bristle.

.... *fifty-eight*

Matt stares out the window. Listless. "I didn't do it, Mike. Why won't they believe me?"

Mike listens. Patient. "You were despondent. And there's no evidence otherwise. How did the poison get in the food if you didn't put it there?"

Matt watches nothing. Numb.

"Who was in the house that day, Matt?"

"Just me. And Alex's friend."

"Alex's friend?"

"Kevin."

Mike's eyes. Surprise. "What was he doing there?"

"He came by to tell me he'd seen Alex. And she wanted him to come by. Tell me she was okay. I figured Alex told you."

Mike's eyes narrow. "No. She didn't."

Matt doesn't move.

"Maybe he did it." Mike walks and talks. "Obsession. With Alex."

Matt. No emotion. "Sooner or later. It happens to everyone. With her."

Alex drives beneath the blood red moon.

She looks in the rearview.

A motorcycle gains on her.

Chills.

Pulls up to the driver's side. Keeps pace with her.

The driver stares at her behind the helmet.
She can't see his face.
Try to breathe Alex. Your heart's in your ears.
The rider salutes. Zooms off.
Alex pulls to the side of the road.
Abrupt.
Gasps.

Matt stares at a sketch of Alex amidst a sea of shiny wrappers.

No face. Only wings.

The orderly brings him the mail.

An envelope.

From Mexico.

He pulls out the picture of Kevin and Alex from years ago. Turns it over.

"Alex blackmailed me into poisoning you. I think she wants me dead too. She already tried once. If I don't make it back from Mexico check the glove compartment. Kevin."

Matt's eyes.

Burn.

Alex enters. "Matt, I'm sorry I couldn't get by here before."

He slides the picture under his robe. Doesn't turn to look at her. "Where were you?"

Alex paces. Searches for a cigarette. The pack is empty. "I went down to Mexico. On a job."

"Run into Kevin? He said he was going down there."

Alex. Nervous. "No. I didn't. See him." She watches a big woman slapping a little man in the parking lot.

"Too bad."

"Mike's gonna get you out of here, Matt. I promise."

"Maybe Kevin put the poison in my food, Alex. Maybe he has an obsession with you."

He turns and stares at her. Through her. She shivers.

"You're the only one with the obsession, Matt. You have to let it go."

She disappears.

He pulls out the picture.

Tears.

He dials.

"There's something I want to show you, Mike."

.... *fifty-nine*

The flashlight beam hits the glove compartment.
Mike opens it.
The poison bottle inside.
He puts it in a plastic bag.
He already knows her prints are on it.
He looks up at Norma's room. The warm light inside.

Alex reads the end of the book. "'The Wild Things roared their terrible roars and gnashed their terrible teeth and rolled their terrible eyes and showed their terrible claws but Max stepped into his private boat and waved good-bye. And sailed back over a year and in and out of weeks and through a day and into the night of his very own room where he found his supper waiting. And it was still hot.'"

She puts the book down. Kisses Norma Jean.

"Okay. Sleep tight."

"Why were they going to eat him up if he didn't stay?"

"They said because they loved him. But that's not a good kind of love, baby."

"Why did they want to hurt Max if they loved him?"

"People just do that sometimes, baby. I don't know why."

"Mama, when I grow up. I want to be the 'wildest one of all'. Like Max." Her strong little eyes flash.

Alex hugs her. "Just always be yourself, baby. Always be Norma Jean."

Alex goes to the door.

"When will Daddy come home, Mama?"

Guilt. "I don't know, baby. Soon."

"I love you , Mama."

"I love you too, baby."

The small pool of light hits the lab report on Mike's desk. Same poison used to drug Matt.

He stares at the picture of Kevin and Alex.

Their embrace.

The lies.

.... *sixty*

"Can I come in?" Mike stands on the doorstep. Sober.

"Why are you being so polite?" Alex waves him in. Suspicious. "What? What's wrong?"

"Tell me what happened in Mexico."

Alex looks for a cigarette. Away from his eyes.

Fingers fidget. "I told you. No point in talking about that."

"Where's Kevin, Alex?"

"Gone." She finds one. Lights it.

"How far did the game go down there? How far did YOU go?" Accusing.

"What are you saying, Mike?" Disappointed.

"All I need is a straight answer."

Their eyes.

Her smoke.

"I'm going down there, Alex. To get some straight answers from Kevin."

"You can't." Fingers play with the cigarette. "He's gone."

Mike jerks the door open. Betrayed. "I'll find him."

Alex follows him out the door.

"Why are you doing this?"

He gets in the Porsche. No answer.

"Mike. Can't you just. Trust me."

The door slams.

He peels out.

Their eyes.

.... *sixty-one*

The patrol officer allows Alex south of the border.

The convertible speeds down the highway.

Marilyn flaps in the breeze.

Alex. Stone face.

Desperate.

Her headlight beams bob up to the ravine.

She stays in the car.

Remembers.

Finally climbs out.

To the edge.

Shines a flashlight into the chasm.

The beam travels.

Travels.

Nothing.

Alex waves the flashlight around the space. Frantic.

The motorcycle is gone.

So is the body.

"What are you looking for, Alex. The motorcycle?"

"Shit!" She jumps. Turns.

Mike. A cold stare.

"You scared the hell out of me. What are you doing here?"

She stares at him. It sinks in. "You followed me. You set me up. You son of a bitch. You don't know the whole story."

He toes the tire marks at the edge of the cliff. "Yes. I do. You cut the brake line. You led him here to the edge in a chase.

One of your games. You stopped. He didn't. I leave anything out?"

His icy eyes. She doesn't know this stranger.

"I had to." Pleading.

"Course you did. Because you had him poison Matt."

Alex is stunned. "I didn't tell him to poison Matt. I found the bottle in his duffel bag after I called you from the motel."

"Why didn't you tell me about it, Alex? Why didn't you give it to me? As evidence." He doesn't believe her.

"Because I left it in the motel room when I was running for my fucking life." Smartass. She stares at him. Overwhelmed at this turn. "I can't believe this."

He continues. Unwavering. "The bottle was hidden in your glove compartment, Alex. I found it there."

Her brain swims. "That's impossible."

Mike cuffs her.

"Mike. Please. Listen to me. He's still playing. He had somebody put it there. I didn't try to kill my husband. Don't do this to me. Don't do this to Norma Jean."

Mike drags her to the car. "By the way. All I found was the bike. Where'd you put the body, Alex?"

"Fuck you."

Mike shoves her in the car. "I'm doing you one last favor, doll. I'm taking you back so you can be tried there for attempted murder. Instead of disappearing in some jail down here for homicide."

"You're a real prince, Mike. You know, I thought you were different. Not possessive. Not competitive. I thought you actually had balls. Instead of thinking with them. You want me in a goddamned box." She looks away. Disgust. "You're just like all the rest."

He turns the keys.

His eyes. So cold.

"So are you, sweetheart. So are you."

.... *sixty-two*

Alex rubs her temples in the cell.

Dying for a cigarette.

A guard opens the door. Her lawyer is smiling.

"You made bail."

"How? My father disowned me. Along with everybody else."

The lawyer is confused. "B.B. Jajonavitch. You don't know this B.B.?"

Alex nods. "Never heard of him."

The lawyer leads her out. "Maybe he's one of those people who sees someone's crime picture in the paper and falls in love."

"I don't care. I can see Norma Jean."

The lawyer's smile fades. He stops Alex. "Look. She's. Gone."

Alex spins. "Gone? What do you mean? Gone."

"Your parents."

Alex's brain implodes. Twelve year old memories. Pull up your socks. Nobody wants an ugly girl. Make sure you keep Matt happy. Baby doll.

"My father has no right."

"He does."

This knocks the breath out of Alex.

"Matt?"

The lawyer nods. "You can fight it. I'll be tough."

Alex's eyes. Fire.

"If I'd fought him before. My father. Just once. I wouldn't be here now."

She thinks about a lifetime of bad choices.

"Norma's not gonna be another 'baby doll'."

She slams through the gates.

"Not while I'm breathin'."

They clang.

Ominous.

.... sixty-three

The convertible pulls up to Corine's. The women hug.

"Oh, honey, I'm so glad you're out." Corine pulls her to the steps.

"I'm going to get Norma."

Corine's smile fades.

"Why you want to go and do that? Your Daddy."

"My Daddy's not raisin' Norma."

"You got no respect, Alex."

"I need some money, Corine. Just a loan."

Corine peeks around for Eddie. "He doesn't know where I keep the tips." She disappears inside. Reappears with a wad of cash.

Alex takes it.

"Don't ask for more trouble than you need, Alex."

"I've been asking for trouble all my life, Corine. And none of it made much of a difference. Men. Highs. Didn't matter. The next day was still there to get through. As me. Only I didn't ever know who that was. I'm not sure I do now. But I'm not who they think I am. I'm through with that. I'm takin' my daughter and we're gonna build something. I don't know what. But we're gonna live without feeling like we can't breathe." Her eyes are lit with new horizons.

Corine doesn't know what to make of that kind of freedom. It's more scary than Eddie's fist.

"You are crazy to try and raise a baby alone, Alex. Crazy."

Alex hugs her. "Good-bye, Corine."

Corine watches her drive off.
Eddie yells.

.... sixty-four

Alex stands before the house. The twelve year old inside stirring.

Her father and mother. And Matt. Stare from the porch. Silence. Judgment.

"Mama!" Norma Jean breaks away from Alex Sr.'s grip and runs to hug Alex. Alex leans down and sweeps Norma into her arms.

Her hope.

"Norma Jean. Baby."

"I missed you, Mama."

I missed you too, baby."

She stares at Matt and her parents over Norma's shoulder.

"But we'll be able to see each other now."

Alex Sr. calls from the porch. "Norma! Norma Jean! Time to wash for dinner."

Norma looks at him. At Alex. Torn. "Did you really hurt Daddy?"

"I wasn't very nice to your Daddy. But I didn't try to hurt him. No matter what anybody says, baby."

Norma fiddles with her hair. "Did you really hurt that man?"

Alex sighs. "I just wasn't very smart, baby. I wasn't. Smart."

Her father on the steps. Disapproving.

Alex's eyes. His eyes.

She takes Norma's hand. "You heard him. Time to wash for dinner."

She stares into his eyes. Makes the long walk across the yard. Unwavering.

Alex lets go of Norma's hand as they reach the steps.

Alex Sr. pats her head. "Go on. Baby doll."

Alex leans down to kiss her. "You're gonna stay with Grampa and Grandma for a little while. But I'm coming back for you. I promise."

She stands. Looks into her father's eyes. "I'm her mother."

"You're undisciplined. You conduct yourself like a gypsy. You have no roots. No respect."

Alex smiles. Clear. For the first time. "I've spent my entire life trying to prove to you I'm good." She turns to go. "Well I am good. And I don't have to prove that to you. Or another goddamned soul."

She gets in her car. Matt follows after. "Alex…I'll drop the charges. If you'll just. Come home."

She shakes her head. Beyond words.

"We never had a home, Matt. We had a marriage. There's a difference."

His eyes.

A tear.

.... *sixty-five*

Alex sits in the hotel room.
The neon hotel sign flickers stories below.
On.
Off.
On.
Marilyn watches over her on the tube.
The ashes fall on her thighs. Still hot.
She doesn't feel it.
Marilyn gets hit on in a bar.
"Eye contact."
The neon reflects in her eyes.
"That's the whole damn problem."

Matt shuffles through mounds of silver candy wrappers in the house. Drinking.

Meticulously dusts the wedding painting. Now macabre in the shadows.

Suddenly puts a fist through it. Tortured.

Tears.

He falls to his knees.

Wrenching scream.

"It's B.B. Open up."

A wispy black chick stuffs a bail slip through the crack in the door. "She'd better not skip or your ass is grass. Look, I say live and let live and all but you mind telling me why you're letting go of ten big ones for her? She that good a screw?"

The door opens wider. "To screw or be screwed. That is the eternal question."

Kevin flashes a lazy grin.

A tooth is gone.

He closes the door.

A limp.

.... *sixty-six*

The phone rings in the hotel room. Alex wakes up. Disoriented.

Ring.

Ring.

She finally remembers where she is.

And why.

She picks up. "Hello?"

Nothing.

"Hello?"

Breathing. A familiar whisper. "Just wanted to say. I win."

Click. Kevin grins from the phone booth.

She drops the phone.

Backs against the wall.

Looks for her keys.

Can't find them.

Tears the room apart.

Finally grabs them.

Runs for the door.

Siren fingernails reach for the knob.

One long terrifying headlight beam in the window.

She backs away.

Spins.

The window.

Escape.

Can't get it open.

Hurry.

Finally. It acquiesces.
Alex spills out of the hotel room.
Panic.
Down. Blocked.
Up. Intimidating climb.
She hears the door knob turning.
Bolts up.
Heart in her throat.
Looking down the ground tilts.
His hands on the sill. Still coming after her.
She looks back up.
Grabs for the roof.
Swings up to safety. Looks around. No options.
Runs to the edge.
Dizzy.
Tilt.
Runs for the other edge. Contemplating the next roof.
She can make it. Not too far.
Suddenly a familiar voice. Cutting through her.
Startling her. She jerks toward the voice.
"Angel…" Matt is coming towards her. Afraid.
Reaching for her. Desperate to save her.
But the abyss of the night has already grabbed her.
Locked on.
Pulling her backwards.
Their eyes.
Full of the knowledge of the fall.
Its completeness. Its finiteness. Its irony.
"Allie, no, I can't do this without you…"
His hand. Reaching into the nothingness.
Missing her.
The terrible thud.
His face drains.

He sinks to the edge.
A wounded animal.
"No...Angel...I'm...sorry..."
Sobs.
Spent.
He rises.
Looks out at the emptiness.
Spreads his arms. Just like an angel.
Lifts his face to the night.
Falls forward.
After her.

.... *sixty-seven*

A red stoplight.
Traffic criss-crossing.
Kevin grins. Guns it. Screams through the red light.
A car skids to miss him.
Inside the car, Mike. Grim.
On his way to the accident.
Kevin pops off his helmet. Locks eyes with Mike.
Salutes him. Eerie.
Mike. Stunned.
He stops. Looks back after the motorcycle.
Disappearing into the night horizon.
Blank.
Unbelieving.
The puzzle suddenly painfully clear. Irony overwhelming.

.... *sixty-eight*

Mike arrives at the hotel. Marilynesque women tower above the busy crime scene. Omnipotent billboard.

Mike weaves through the stale crime scene.

Cops drink coffee. Laughing.

Coroner makes notes. A crack about Romeo and Juliet.

They stop when Mike passes.

Sober truth on their faces.

In the silence he pauses by Matt's truck.

Lone broken headlight.

The cop pulls the blanket away from the two forms.

Face down. Face up.

Still at sixes and sevens.

"Somebody's gotta tell Norma." The cop half whispers.

Mike's eyes. Full of remorse.

Devastated.

The Marilyn eyes tower over his shoulder.

Smiling.

Blowing a kiss at the bloody scene.

A city full of Normas.

And Marilyns.

the end